Underst
Infant Coil

An Osteopathic Perspective

Clive Hayden MSc, DO, MSCC

Contents

Introduction

When a baby seems to be suffering from digestive difficulties, it can be very difficult to know exactly what is wrong and how to help. It is very distressing to parents if their otherwise happy baby is crying in pain for long periods.

Deciding how best to help the baby is made more difficult because of the multitude of often contradictory and confusing advice offered by everyone – including family, friends and health professionals.

Most people assume that any crying baby is suffering from infantile colic. In reality, there are several different causes of infant digestive disorders, each needing slightly different management.

A crying baby may have no problem with his digestion, but simply be complaining of being uncomfortable somewhere else in his or her body. This is often in the head and neck as a result of being squeezed and twisted during the birth process.

This booklet explains the different causes of colic, and how they are best managed or treated.

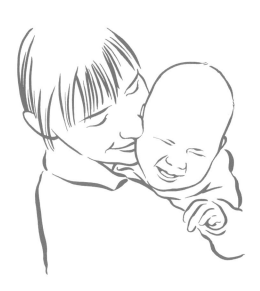

What is infantile colic?

Colic is the general name given to a range of infant digestive disorders, not a single condition. It includes several different types of digestive problems:

- **Reflux**
- **Infant gut irritability**
- **Lactose intolerance**
- **Allergy**

Each of these types of colic has different signs and symptoms, and needs to be managed or treated in different ways. Therefore it is helpful for us to be able to distinguish between them. There may sometimes be a 'blurred picture' with more than one of these types of colic occurring at the same time.

One thing these conditions all have in common is that they are rarely pathological i.e. a disease process is rarely identified. Most of the infants also continue to put on weight, despite the apparent disturbance to their digestive processes. So parents can be reassured that there is little likelihood that their infant is suffering from a serious illness.

Signs and symptoms of colic

- The earliest sign of colic is that the baby is very **flatulent** (farty), and the stools are explosively delivered
- The baby is obviously **uncomfortable** and often seems in considerable **pain**
- The **stomach is distended** or swollen and **loud gurgling** sounds can be heard in the abdomen
- The baby may **arch his back** during a colic attack, and bring his **knees up** to his stomach
- The baby is obviously in pain and may **cry inconsolably** for several hours, and nothing seems to pacify him/her
- The baby may also suffer from low level colic, when he is **restless and uncomfortable** but not crying.

Facts about colic

Colic is the most common and sometimes the most distressing affliction of young infants, affecting up to 30% of babies. Some colicky babies may be more affected than others, and it may lead to bouts of crying, in which the baby cannot be comforted by any means.[1]

Research has shown that approximately half of affected babies improve naturally by 3 months, and by 6 months nearly 9 out of 10 babies have improved, but some infants still have persistent symptoms after this age.[1]

Signs of colic may start soon after birth, but rarely after the first month. At 6-8 weeks after the birth the symptoms seem to peak. Generally those infants that display the earliest symptoms will be the ones most severely affected.

Stress that affects the mother in pregnancy, during labour or after the birth, has also been shown to be a cause of infantile colic.[2, 6]

Research studies have shown that if a baby suffers from severe colic then other brothers and sisters are more likely to be affected.[2] Some races such as the Afro-Caribbean races are also more commonly affected.[3] When these two factors are considered together, it seems that there is also a possible genetic component to infantile colic.

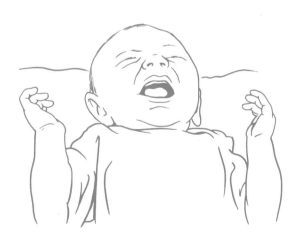

Reflux

Baby cries and grimaces immediately on feeding or within the first 20 minutes

Reflux is when the valve that shuts off the entrance to the stomach fails to work properly and some of the stomach acids escape into the lower part of the oesophagus (which takes the food from the mouth to the stomach). This causes **pain or a burning sensation** (like heartburn). It is often accompanied by **posseting**, when the baby will spit up small amounts of semi-digested milk.

As a personal observation, the infant will almost always grimace and start to cry while feeding or within the first 20 minutes of feeding. Sometimes the baby may have a preferred feeding position – on one particular breast, or resting along one arm, which helps it to be more comfortable.

The **diaphragm** is a dome-shaped sheet of muscle separating the abdomen and chest. It helps to close off the top of the stomach.

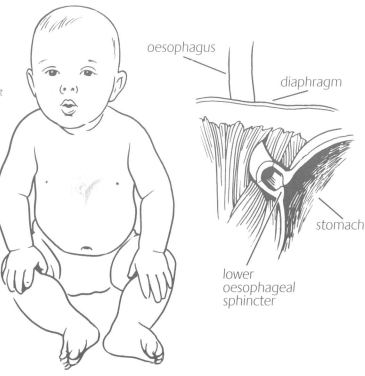

oesophagus

diaphragm

stomach

lower oesophageal sphincter

Possible causes	Leakage of stomach contents is normally prevented by the combined action of an internal valve, with external reinforcement from the fibres of the diaphragm that loop around the lower oesophagus. If the diaphragm is distorted it can disrupt the external muscular component of the sphincter.

As an osteopath I am aware of the twists and strains that affect the infant, many of which have been imposed on the infant by the pressures of birth. Some twists may be due to the infant lying in an awkward way in the womb. I frequently find that reflux in the baby is associated with pressure that was put on the shoulders or rib cage during the delivery. This pressure seems to distort the rib cage, twisting the diaphragm and disrupting the cardiac sphincter.[13]

Management of reflux

Feeding
More frequent, smaller feeds may reduce the levels of symptoms, by reducing the volume of milk in the stomach. Sitting the baby upright or more vertically during or after feeds may also help, as may sloping the cot mattress up at the head end.

Medications
Infant Gaviscon is frequently prescribed as a medication, which will help to ease the symptoms. In more severe cases the medication **Domperidone** or **Omeprazole** is prescribed in order to decrease production of stomach acids.

A special 'extra thick' milk formula is also available, that is more likely to remain in the stomach rather than leaking out into the oesophagus.

Osteopathic treatment

Using gentle osteopathic manipulative techniques, it is possible to release the distortion of the rib cage and thus improve the effectiveness of the sphincter to the stomach. This usually helps the reflux to resolve, although the symptoms rarely resolve immediately. It takes a time for the irritation and sensitivity in the lower part of the oesophagus, caused by burning from stomach acids, to settle. However within a week of the ribcage being treated and 'balanced', the symptoms would usually be expected to ease or show signs of improvement.

Infant gut irritability

Colic symptoms and crying start approximately 30–90 minutes after a feed

From personal observation, this is one of the major causes of colic in infants. The stomach seems to empty too rapidly, moving undigested milk through the small intestine at a great speed. This rapid intestinal movement causes the loud gurgling sounds that are commonly heard. The fermentation of the undigested milk causes the gut to expand which stimulates its contraction further (causing loud stomach sounds) and the pressure in the colon causes pain and eventually explosive flatulence.

Small white flecks of undigested milk may be seen at times in the faeces of the baby (like grains of white rice), especially where the milk has passed through the entire digestive system extremely rapidly. These flecks may also be seen in the faeces of babies who suffer from lactose intolerance.

Management of infant gut irritability

Medications

Some medications such as **infacol** may help this type of colic by slowing down the motion of the intestines. There appears to be variability in the response of infants to **infacol**.

Gripe water is a remedy that has been around for many years – the active component was thought to be alcohol (which is no longer added to gripe water). However it does seem to help some infants.

The pharmaceutical preparation of the lactase enzyme **Colief** may also help by assisting in the digestion of the milk, even when it is suspected that the baby is not lactose intolerant and can digest milk. **Colief** must be given to the baby approximately half an hour before the feed for maximum benefit, making it difficult for parents to predict the timing if the infant is being breastfed on demand. It is perhaps easier to plan when to give **Colief** to a bottle-fed baby.

Possible causes and osteopathic treatment

1. Retained moulding pressure from birth

From my own 31 years experience in working with babies suffering from colic it seems that the irritability of the intestines is part of a stress response of the brain to pressure. This can cause an over excitability of the sympathetic nervous system that manages the internal organs of the body, and increases the activity of the gut.

For the majority of infants who suffer from this bowel irritability, the pressure on the brain will have been caused by the moulding pressure on the baby's head during the birth process. Infants delivered via forceps or ventouse are particularly vulnerable to these pressures. This compression of the cranium doesn't always resolve in the days after birth, especially where the birth has been difficult and traumatic, so the reactivity of the sympathetic nervous system continues. Quick deliveries may also cause a degree of irritation and overstimulation of the nervous system that persists long after birth.

The pressure that I talk about here is not the same as the **medical alert of raised intracranial pressure**.[14] This is where there is a build up of pressure within the skull cavity, either in the fluid (the CSF) that supports and surrounds the brain or when caused by a bleed or haemorrhage within the skull. Rather this pressure that I mention seems to be a response of the delicate nervous system to a mechanical irritation or crowding by the surrounding supportive membranes and bones of the cranium.

For the osteopath it is important to release the tensions and pressures in the cranium that may still be present from the birth, and that may affect the infant's delicate nervous system. These tensions and pressures may also be present even after a caesarean birth especially if the mother has spent some time in normal labour before the caesarean section.

The cranial approach to treatment is very gentle, and works in a way that encourages the tissues to ease and release their own strain patterns, rather than using any strongly applied forces in treatment. This allows the nervous system to return to a more relaxed state and helps to calm the intestines.

2. Irritation of the nerve to the stomach

For a long time osteopaths have considered that the main nerve, the vagus nerve, that supplies the oesophagus, stomach and upper part of the intestines is vulnerable to compression as it exits out through one of the small holes in the base of the skull.[5] This interference with the vagus nerve is thought to cause the stomach to be more sensitive and reactive, so being another cause of colic. Other nerves that exit the skull adjacent to the vagus nerve are involved with the actions of suckling and swallowing, and irritation of these nerves can make suckling and swallowing difficult and tiring for the baby.

It is thought that the small exit hole (called the jugular foramen), in the base of the skull is particularly vulnerable to distortion when the skull is moulded and squeezed during the birth process. The hole is located at the junction of two cranial bones, and contains two other cranial nerves and the main jugular vein, which drains up to 95% of the blood from the skull.

The infant skull seen from below.

The nerve to the stomach is vulnerable to compression as it passes through the jugular foramen.

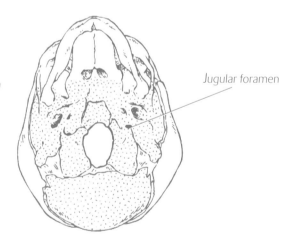

Jugular foramen

Treatment

There are some very effective, specific, but gentle techniques used by osteopaths to release the specific distortion of the jugular foramen.

3. Caesarean birth

Babies born by caesarean section may suffer from infantile colic, but the incidence is lower than in babies born vaginally.[6]

Babies born by **emergency caesarean** due to failure to progress in labour will have experienced labour with its intense contractions. They may have been stuck in the birth canal for some time. It is common to find both moulding compressions and strains in these babies, and as such they are vulnerable to all types of colic in the same way as a baby born vaginally.

Babies born by **elective caesarean** may not have been exposed to the pressure of contractions, but they have different things to deal with. There may be a sense of shock due to the sudden nature of the birth without the stimulation of contractions preceding it, which leaves the nervous system over-reactive. There may also be some moulding compression from being cramped in a confined space during the last few weeks of pregnancy. These may be contributing factors to colic.

Infants born by caesarean who suffer from colic are perhaps more likely than vaginally born babies to be suffering from lactose intolerance, or inability to produce the lactase enzyme necessary to digest the lactose sugars in the milk.[6]

Osteopathic treatment

There is no single prescribed osteopathic treatment or technique for treating babies with colic. Osteopaths work with the whole body to release tensions and stresses wherever they are found, to restore a sense of balance, harmony and relaxation to the whole body. As such each baby may be treated differently, although there are some common findings in colicky babies as described above.

Recent research has demonstrated that osteopathy is highly effective in treating colicky babies.[4] The research results showed that not only did treated infants cry less, but they also showed a significant improvement in hours of restful sleep.

Lactose intolerance

Colicky symptoms tend to occur approximately 2 hours after a feed

The baby lacks the ability to produce the **lactase dehydrogenase enzyme** which is necessary to break down the lactose component of the milk. Therefore the milk moves through the gut without being digested or broken down. It takes approximately two hours for the milk to move out of the stomach, through the small intestine and into the large intestine. The undigested milk then starts to ferment in the large intestine, fairly quickly causing the intestine to distend and swell and the baby to start feeling signs of discomfort and pain.[7] Therefore the colic is usually worst about 2 hours after a feed.

The fermenting milk produces gas which swells the intestines, which in turn is a trigger for increasing the rate of peristalsis in the gut – and the gurgling commences. Peristalsis is the name given to the rhythmical wave of contraction that passes down the intestines, helping to propel the food matter through the gut. The rate can vary from individual to individual, meaning that the gut transit time (the time taken for food to pass through the entire intestinal system) will vary with different people. Stress is also acknowledged as having an effect in speeding up the gut transit time.[2] Increasing the amount of roughage and fibre in the diet can also speed up the gut transit time.

Research into a large group of 9 year-old children found that 24% of children had signs of lactose intolerance.[9] This is a 1:4 ratio and seems quite high. Some Afro-Caribbean races also seem to have a higher tendency than other races to show signs of lactose intolerance.[3]

Family history

There is often a family history, either on the mother's or the father's side of a family member who also dislikes milk. They may not know that they are possibly lactose intolerant but have naturally avoided drinking raw milk, because for them it just seems to sit in the stomach as an undigested mass feeling very uncomfortable. So they have learnt to avoid raw milk – such as on breakfast cereals or a glass of milk. They may decide to have toast and another drink instead for breakfast.

Very often these people can eat cheese and yoghurts, but in these foods the milk is already partially broken down by the process of making the cheese and yoghurts. One of the most popular misunderstandings is that lactose intolerance is an allergic reaction by the baby to the milk. This is simply not true. Lactose intolerance means that the infant cannot produce for itself the enzyme necessary for breaking down the lactose component of milk.

This inability of the infant to produce lactase means that it is unlikely to be able to digest the lactose **in any animal milk**. This includes human breast milk, cows milk and goat's milk. Severely affected infants may well benefit from being fed animal protein-free formula milk. A number of these are available to buy in shops and chemists, or may be prescribed by the doctor.

Management of lactose intolerance

Mother's diet
For a breast fed baby it may help if the mother eliminates all dairy products from her diet.

Medication
The pharmaceutical preparation of the lactase enzyme, **Colief**, may help by assisting in the digestion of the milk. **Colief** must be given to the baby approximately half an hour before the feed for maximum benefit, making it difficult for parents to predict the timing if the infant is being breast-fed on demand.

Osteopathic treatment

It is not possible to directly treat the lactose intolerance with osteopathic treatment. However these babies do often show an improvement in their ability to cope with the digestive difficulties if they receive osteopathic treatment.[4] Osteopathic treatment is aimed at releasing any compressions, strains and twists that may be making them generally more tense and reactive.

These babies may also be suffering from one of the other causes of colic as well as the lactose intolerance. Osteopathic treatment, depending on diagnostic and palpatory findings, may help to treat some of the other conditions that are also affecting the infant. This in turn appears to make the infant more comfortable, helping it to cope better with the discomfort of the lactose intolerant colic.

Allergies

The timing of a reaction is less clear cut in relation to feeds. The reaction is more likely soon after a feed.

Signs of allergy

Any or all of these signs may be present

- **Gut discomfort**, no clear-cut timing in relation to feeds
- **Vomiting** small or substantial parts of the feed, often soon after the feed
- Excessive clear **mucous production** in nose and sinuses, which may make the baby sound blocked in the nose and in older children may contribute to middle ear infections
- **Skin reactions**. In my opinion rashes, cradle cap, dry patches of skin and excema are all signs of an allergic response in the baby.

Babies can be allergic to milk or a component of that milk. A cow's milk allergy is a fairly common occurrence in bottle-fed babies.[8] Breastfed babies can react to substances eaten by the mother.

I usually ask the mother:

- If she has any suspicion that any food that she has eaten recently is causing her baby to react?
- If there are any known allergies that affect a member of their near family. This includes dad as well as uncles, aunts, grandparents (of the baby) and any of the baby's siblings (brothers or sisters). If so then I might start to suspect that the infant is also reacting to the same substances.

The challenge test for the breast-fed baby

If the mother suspects that certain foods are upsetting the baby's digestion, I ask her to avoid that food or substance for a week, and monitor the signs of allergy in the infant. Then I suggest that the mother eats that food and observe the reaction in the baby. The reaction may show in the skin, but it can also affect their digestion as well as upsetting their behaviour. It is best that the mother only tests one food or substance at a time, otherwise the whole picture gets confusing. The advantage of adopting this approach is that the mother can be performing some simple screening tests of her own.

Management of allergies

For a breast fed baby, the mother should avoid eating foods that may be causing the baby to react.

For a bottle fed baby, there are certain non-animal preparations of milk that may be helpful. These are available either to buy over the counter, or on prescription for severely affected infants.

There are various skin tests that may be performed in special hospital clinics to determine the nature of the allergy. Other blood tests have been shown to be extremely reliable because repeat testing of blood samples demonstrates a high level of consistency with the results. Tests may also be performed on a hair sample, and the examination and culture of the faeces may also indicate possibilities of identifying the cause of the reaction in the infant.

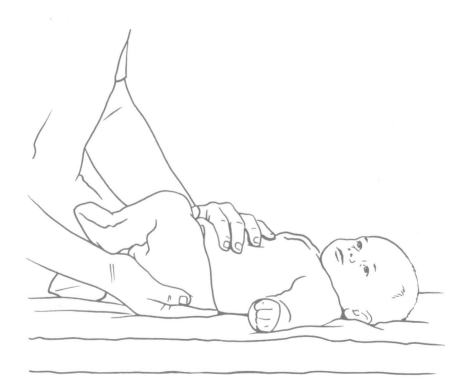

Summary of colic

A baby may suffer from more than one cause of colic, which can present a confusing picture. There may be any combination of reflux (pain soon after a feed), gut irritability (pain 30 to 90 minutes after a feed), and lactose intolerance (pain about two hours after a feed). It may seem that the digestive discomfort is present all the time and does not follow any timing pattern in relation to feeds, hence different management strategies need to be tried in order to find the best approach for that particular baby.

Crying baby

No relation to feeding

No abdominal signs, sickness etc

Associated with feeding

Abdominal signs

Reflux 0–20 minutes	**Gut irritability** 30–90 minutes	**Lactose intolerance** 2+ hours
Cries on feeding. Posseting. No explosive nappies or other abdominal signs.	Distended abdomen. Loud gurgling stomach. Explosive nappies.	Explosive nappies. Other abdominal signs.

Unsettled, irritable baby

May be uncomfortable somewhere else. Often from birth compression.

Treatment	**Treatment**	**Treatment**
Gaviscon Omeprazole Domperidome Osteopathy	Infacol Gripe water Osteopathy	Colief Osteopathy

Osteopathic treatment

To release birth strains and relax the baby

Osteopathic treatment	**Osteopathic treatment**	**Osteopathic treatment**
To release twist in ribcage and diaphragm	To settle irritable cranium and relax tense, irritable infant	To ease stomach congestion and relax tense, irritable infant

Happy, settled infant

Happier (but not totally settled) infant

Sickness and vomiting

Babies are often sick, and this can vary from a small posset of overflow milk, to the gushing vomit of a whole feed.

There are many different causes of vomiting and sickness, for example:

Baby vomits small quantities of milk after feeds

Overfeeding – Infants do not necessarily have a problem if they have just vomited. All infants may be sick at some time, especially if they have overfed (greedy babies do this frequently!). Their stomachs at day 1 are the size of a large marble, at day 3 the size of a ping-pong ball, and at day 10 the size of a chicken's egg.[12] This means that they simply do not have enough space at times in their stomachs to hold much food.

With burping – An infant may posset when it is winded and burped, i.e. the air in the stomach may push up some recently ingested food. This is quite normal and is to be expected from time to time.

Reflux – Infants who suffer from reflux will invariably posset soon after a feed, i.e. spit up small amounts of fairly fresh milk. A burp isn't necessarily an accompaning part of posseting. This is usually accompanied by crying from the baby as the acidified milk irritates and burns the sensitive lower end of the oesophageal tube taking food from the mouth to the stomach.

Colic – True colic, with the loud stomach signs and explosive flatulence, and where reflux is not suspected, is rarely accompanied by vomiting. This is not an absolute rule, as there may frequently be a mix of different conditions.

Baby vomits whole feeds

Allergy – A baby may be reacting to a constituent of the milk, as an allergic response. Some external signs such as rashes on the skin of the baby would usually accompany this gushing vomit. I feel the infant's stomach is literally rejecting the feed. With the breast-fed infant, there might be some variability with the vomiting i.e. the baby may vomit some feeds and not others (partly because the constituents of breast milk will depend on the normal variability in the mother's diet). It is perhaps easier to determine whether a bottle-fed infant is allergic to the type of formula ie cow's milk, or goat's milk, because switching to a different type of formula may soon alter the sickness symptoms.

Pyloric stenosis – Infants who sick up copious amounts of feed some time after the feed may be suffering from pyloric stenosis. The pyloric sphincter is the valve or sphincter that shuts off the exit of the stomach. It opens to let the partially digested food drain from the stomach into the small intestines. Sometimes the muscles in this exit valve can go into spasm, preventing the stomach from emptying. Eventually the body chooses to expel this food from the stomach by vomiting – but it all comes up and can be quite smelly, and curdled. The vomiting may also be seemingly projectile – or can gush a long way, and be very messy! Changes of clothes for the baby are often a necessity!

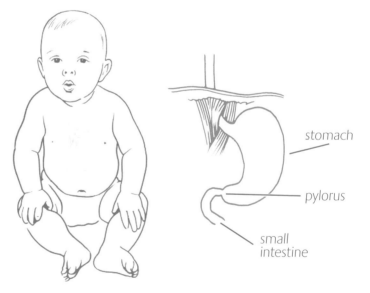

The **pyloric sphincter** closes the lower end of the stomach.

stomach

pylorus

small intestine

The puzzling aspect is that not every feed will be vomited in this way – there is a variability that is difficult to explain. Although the vomit will gush from the infant it is not essentially projectile, and this may be a way of distinguishing pyloric stenosis from the more medically serious 'raised intracranial pressure'. If the pyloric stenosis is severe the baby will usually lose weight, and an operation to release the contractured pyloric sphincter muscles may be necessary. The pylorus can be palpated or felt, as a walnut-shaped lump through the abdominal wall, especially when in spasm.

Projectile vomiting – True projectile vomiting may be indicative of a more serious medical condition of **raised intracranial pressure**. Vomit can literally be ejected from the baby for quite a distance. This is a serious state (but thankfully fairly rare) in which the fluid that supports the delicate brain and nervous system has increased in pressure. If your baby does display projectile vomiting, **it is essential that your doctor be consulted without delay** because this may well be a **medical emergency**.

Blockage within the intestines – Occasionally infants may have a blockage, partial blockage or narrowing in part of their intestinal system.[15]

The **full blockage** or atresia, will prevent the feed from passing down the intestines, and perhaps several hours after a feed it will be ejected. It will look quite dark and be quite smelly. The baby will inevitably lose weight rapidly. Every feed will eventually be vomited. Faeces will be absent or extremely limited.

A **partial blockage** or stricture, may allow the passage of some of the feed, with the faeces being small and scanty in character. There may also be vomiting of the backed up feed that cannot pass through the intestines. This vomit will also be smelly and dark in character. Depending on the severity of the stricture the baby will also lose weight, but less quickly than with a full atresia.

Summary of causes of vomiting

Reflux – Small amounts of posset, usually with the feed. Some crying.

Allergy – Often large amounts of vomit. Variable. Usually with skin rashes or dryness.

Pyloric stenosis – Large amounts of partially digested feed. Variable. Pylorus can be palpated.

Projectile vomiting – **A medical emergency**. Vomit may be ejected quite a distance.

Atresia or stricture – Every feed vomited. Baby loses weight. Vomit is smelly and dark.

How to help your baby cope with colic

Specific management for different types of colic has been discussed in the relevant sections.

However, there are some general things that parents can do to help their colicky baby:

Clothing
It is best to avoid baby clothes with elasticated waists that can put pressure on a bloated and painful stomach.

Feeds should be at least 3 hours apart
When a baby is unsettled or crying, it is tempting to offer them food to try to pacify them. However if your baby is suffering from colic, then it means that he is still struggling to digest the previous feed. Offering him more feed will only make matters worse. It is therefore important that feeds should be at least 3 hours apart.

Winding after feeds
Trapped wind in the stomach may well make a baby uncomfortable. It does help to reduce colic if the baby can bring up trapped wind after feeding, to try to reduce the amount of air in the digestive system. However in colic babies, most of the painful wind is produced by fermentation of the milk lower down in the intestines so burping on its own will not prevent colic.

Babies who struggle to bring up wind after a feed often have tension in the diaphragm. This can be caused by the twisting and turning of the rib cage under compression as it passes through the birth canal. This problem is usually resolved with osteopathic treatment.

Easing reflux symptoms
- It is sometimes better to feed an infant with reflux more frequently. Little and often can help
- Feeding the baby whilst holding it in a more upright position either when breast or bottle-fed may also help
- Keep the baby upright for 30 minutes after a feed

- When laying the baby down, raise the head end of the mattress – perhaps by putting a folded towel or small cushion under the mattress.

Baby massage
Anything that helps the baby to remain relaxed and calm may help him to cope with colic. So gentle massage, of the whole body not just the stomach, may help. This is best done when the baby is quiet or only mildly uncomfortable. If the baby is really upset and crying or screaming due to colic, massage is unlikely to help at this stage.

Breastfed babies – Mother's diet
Brassicas Most infants find it difficult to digest the brassica family of vegetables. These are **broccoli**, **cabbage**, **cauliflower, brussel sprouts** and **lettuce**. These contain natural alkaloids that babies struggle to digest and also find quite bitter to taste.

Bananas can also be difficult to digest. Bananas are high in complex carbohydrates that are more difficult to break down and digest. They are also high in potassium and contain natural adrenalin and dopamines, which can excite the infant and affect the contraction of their muscles.

Very spicy foods can also upset the babies' digestion.

Caffeine It is also wise to avoid drinking too much caffeine, which is a stimulant to both mother and baby. This includes **caffeinated coffee, tea**, and **caffeinated soft drinks**. Some **chocolate** also has a high level of caffeine and other stimulants that can be passed through to the breast fed baby.

For lactose intolerant babies it may help for the mother to avoid eating **dairy products**.

Bottle fed babies
There is an enormous choice of baby milks on the market, and it can be tempting to keep changing the type of milk to find one that helps the colic. It takes several days for a baby to adjust to a different milk formula, and as there can be a number of other variables as well, it can be difficult to know whether it is the change of milk that is helping the baby. As a rule, it is best not

to change the milk formula unless nothing else has helped, and certainly not to keep changing to different milk formulae.

There are a number of 'easy digest' formulas available commercially which may ease the symptoms of colic. These have been partially hydrolysed (i.e. broken down), making them easier to digest, and may well be worth trying.

Medication

Colic has many causes, and medications will more often ease the symptoms rather than cure them. Unless stated, all the following medications are available to buy over the counter in chemists.

Infacol is an anti-spasmodic medication (i.e. it slows down the motion of the gut) that may alleviate some of the symptoms of colic. Not all infants will benefit from it, and the evidence is not clear that it is more effective than a placebo.

Gripe water is a remedy that has been around for many years – the active component was thought to be alcohol (which is no longer added to gripe water). However it does seem to help some infants.

Colief (the pharmaceutical preparation of the lactase enzyme) will often help babies who suffer from lactose intolerance. Indeed a beneficial response to the colief may help to confirm that the baby may be lactose intolerant.

Reflux Medications that help the symptoms of reflux appear to fall into 2 categories.

1. **Infant Gaviscon** is an antacid that reduces the acidity of the stomach secretions, making the gastric juices less likely to burn the oesophageal tissues in the tube leading to the entrance of the stomach. Infant Gaviscon is available to buy over the counter or is prescribed by doctors.

2. Others such as **Domperidone** and **Omeprazole** will suppress or reduce the amount of acid produced in the stomach. All appear to be effective in easing the symptoms of reflux, but if the reflux is due to the valve at the entrance to the stomach not closing properly, they will not solve this problem. These medications are only available on prescription.

Osteopathic treatment

Osteopathy is often effective at relieving the symptoms of Infantile Colic. Osteopaths treat the whole body of the baby to relieve and release any areas of tension.

Particular attention is paid to

- The **head**, that is subjected to large compressive forces during labour, which can leave it distorted or compressed
- The **diaphragm** which is so important for the stomach, both in allowing the baby to bring up wind after a feed, and in shutting off the entrance to the stomach to prevent reflux. Twisting forces through the rib cage during birth (particularly in posterior presentations where the baby turns through 270 degrees within the birth canal) can distort the diaphragm and sphincter to the stomach
- The **gut** itself can also be treated to relax the muscles in the wall of the gut, so calming the irritability.

Osteopathic treatment of babies is very gentle. They usually enjoy their treatment and often fall asleep during or after it.

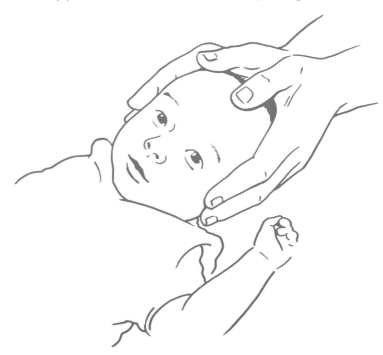

Colic – Frequently asked questions

Is breast milk easier for my baby to digest than formula milk?

There is very little evidence to suggest that this is the case. However it is thought that human breast milk proteins are more naturally compatible with the infant digestive processes. Breast milk has many other advantages for the developing infant, particularly in helping develop a healthy immune system.

Are any therapies effective in treating colic, and what evidence is there to justify the claims made?

A small cranial osteopathic research study comparing 14 treated infants with 14 controls was published in 2006.[4] The results showed that osteopathy is very effective at relieving symptoms of colic, and a larger scale research study is currently being planned. There are several published studies on the benefits of chiropractic treatment.

Some homoeopathic remedies have been found to work although there does not appear to be any published research material available. Reflexology also claims to help, but there is little evidence to back this up. Infant massage can also help to relax and settle the baby as pain and discomfort will make the baby tense, and anything that helps to relax the baby is worth trying.

What is the difference between infant gut irritability and lactose intolerance?

Lactose intolerance differs from infant gut irritability because in lactose intolerance the baby cannot produce enough of the enzyme necessary to digest the milk, so milk passes through the gut undigested. In infant gut irritability the baby can produce the enzyme but the milk passes through the gut too quickly for the enzyme to be able to work properly. In both conditions the end result is the same, the fermentation of the milk in the large intestine producing wind and hence colic.

Will my baby's symptoms disappear by 3 months?

For a long time it was thought that the symptoms of colic disappeared by the age of 3 months – and the condition was labelled '3-month colic'.[10] In 1983 a study of 983 colicky infants found that 47% of these infants improved by 3 months; 41% improved by 6 months, leaving the symptoms of the remaining 12% going on after 6 months of age.[11]

Therefore it seems that nearly half of infants will improve by 3 months, but for the rest their symptoms may persist for quite some time.

Why are the symptoms often worse in the evening?	The same study in 1983 [11] also found that only 1 in 4 infants (24%) showed signs of being worse in the evening. In my opinion though, symptoms that get worse in the evening are often due to the baby becoming tired and irritable as the day progresses, and getting more upset by the time evening comes.

Commonly given advice is to try to avoid over-stimulating and overtiring the baby. It may help to reduce the number of visitors during the day, and avoid an over busy lifestyle i.e. to try to keep the baby as calm as possible.

It may also signify to me that the infant is more likely to have been affected by musculo-skeletal strains (probably acquired during the birth process), and that this is the probable cause of their colic. The effect of the tension in the baby is to make them more tired by the end of the day.

Is my colicky baby allergic to milk?	Research has shown [3] that colicky babies are no more likely to be allergic to milk than all the other babies. However, in my opinion, the skin is often the best indicator of allergic reactions. Rashes, cradle cap and dry patches of skin may be an indication of an allergy to a substance in the milk.

The baby who pulls away from the breast whilst feeding, crying in discomfort, is more likely to be suffering from the pain of reflux than being allergic to the milk. Some mothers who observe their baby supposedly grimacing when starting to feed, think that the baby doesn't like the taste of the milk or is reacting to it. More often than not it is the discomfort of reflux that makes them do that.

If I have any more children, will they also be more likely to be affected?	Unfortunately for you, research evidence has found that when you have had one baby who suffered from colic, any other children you have are more likely to be affected.[1] This does not mean that you will definitely have another baby who suffers from colic – but it is more likely.

In my opinion this suggests that the cause is more likely to be lactose intolerance, which is likely to be an inherited or genetic condition. When traumatic birth factors seem to be the major cause, it may well be that the first-born is more likely to be the baby most affected.[2] This may be due to the mother's first labour often being longer and more difficult, with subsequent labours often (but not always) being easier and quicker.

Are we doing anything wrong in our care of our baby?

Caring for a distressed, crying infant who cannot be soothed or comforted will challenge the parenting and caring skills of almost all parents. It is a powerful instinct to care and protect our children, and an inability to do this may make any normal person feel inadequate. It is therefore important to understand that your baby is not just being difficult, and that it is possible to understand why they are so upset – and what the possible remedies and treatments are. What is also important is that you try and seek appropriate professional help, and do not feel that you have to cope with your baby on your own. While it may seem a complicated process trying to work out what is the problem with your infant, there are clues (mentioned in earlier texts) that we can use to understand their condition better – and then to try and help them.

What happens to the birth strains if my child does not receive osteopathic treatment?

It is certainly true that colic symptoms do improve eventually, even in the most persistent cases. However many toddlers and young children do suffer from 'tummy aches' especially if stressed or anxious, and it is interesting to wonder whether this is a similar type of condition as infant colic.

If left untreated the birth strain patterns persist as the child grows and can cause a number of other problems later on. These include difficulty sleeping, behavioural problems, ear infections and glue ear, sinus problems, concentration difficulties, poor posture, headaches, and many other problems.

Osteopaths recommend that all babies are checked to release any physical strains caused by the pregnancy and birth, to try to prevent problems later on.

References

1. Stahlberg MR. Infantile Colic: occurrence and risk factors. Eur J Paediatr 1984;143(2):108-11.

2. Rautava P., Lehtonen L., Psychosocial predisposing factors for Infantile Colic. BMJ 1993, 307 pp600-4.

3. Liebman W., Infantile Colic: Association with Lactose and Milk Intolerance. Jama Feb 20, 1981. vol 245, no.7.

4. Hayden C., Mullinger B., A preliminary assessment of the impact of cranial osteopathy for the relief of infantile colic. Complement Ther Clin Pract 2006;12(2):83-90.

5. Magoun H., Osteopathy in the Cranial Field, 3rd edition, chapter 11, p228.

6. Hogdall C., Vestermak V., Birch M., et al. The significancy of pregnancy, delivery and post-partum factors for the development of infantile colic. Journal Perinat Med 19 (1991) pp251-257.

7. Marieb E., Human Anatomy and Physiology, 4th edition. 1998. Pub Benjamin Cummings.

8. Hill D., Hudson I., Sheffield L., et al. A low allergen diet is a significant intervention in Infantile Colic: Results in a community based survey. J Allergy Clin Immunol 1995 vol 56, no.6, part 1.

9. Webster R., DiPalma J., Gremse D., Lactose Maldigestion and Recurrent Abdominal Pain in Children. Digestive Dis and Science. July 1995. Vol 40. no 7. pp1506-1510.

10. Illingworth R.S., Three-Month Colic. Arch Dis Child. Jan 15th 1954. pp165-174.

11. Hide D., Guyer B., Prevalance of Infantile Colic. Arch Dis Child. 1982. pp559-560.

12. Linda J Smith (Coach's notebook: Games and strategies for lactation education) Boston Jones and Bartlett 2002.

13. Serguff N. Cranial Osteopathy for Infants, Children and Adolescents pp278-281, Churchill Livingston Elsevier.

14. Behrman R., Kliegman R., Nelson Essentials of Paediatrics 3rd Edition. p712, W. B. Saunders Company.

15. Carriero, J. An Osteopathic Approach to Children p179. Churchill Livingstone.

Finding a local Osteopath

The contacts below may be useful in helping you to find the nearest osteopath to you specialising in paediatrics. Both the Sutherland Cranial College and Foundation for Paediatric Osteopathy are organisations offering specialist paediatric postgraduate training to qualified osteopaths and as such are well placed to assist you in finding a local osteopath who specialises in this area.

Sutherland Cranial College (SCC)
Tel: 01291 689908
www.sutherlandcranialcollege.co.uk

Osteopathic Centre for Children / Foundation for Paediatric Osteopathy
15a Woodbridge Street, Clerkenwell, London EC1R OND
Tel: 020 7490 5510
www.fco.org.uk

Not all osteopaths specialise in paediatrics. If you are unable to locate a local osteopath from the above organisations, it may be worth finding out about local osteopaths from the General Osteopathic Council or British Osteopathic Association and speaking to the osteopath prior to taking your infant in for treatment.

General Osteopathic Council
Tel: 0207 7357 6655
www.osteopathy.org.uk

British Osteopathic Association
3 Park Terrace, Manor Road, Luton, Beds, LU1 3HN
Tel: 01582 488455
www.osteopathy.org